FASTER
STRONGER
WISER
Faster Stronger Wiser
Jump
Training
WRITTEN BY
Glenn Payne Jr

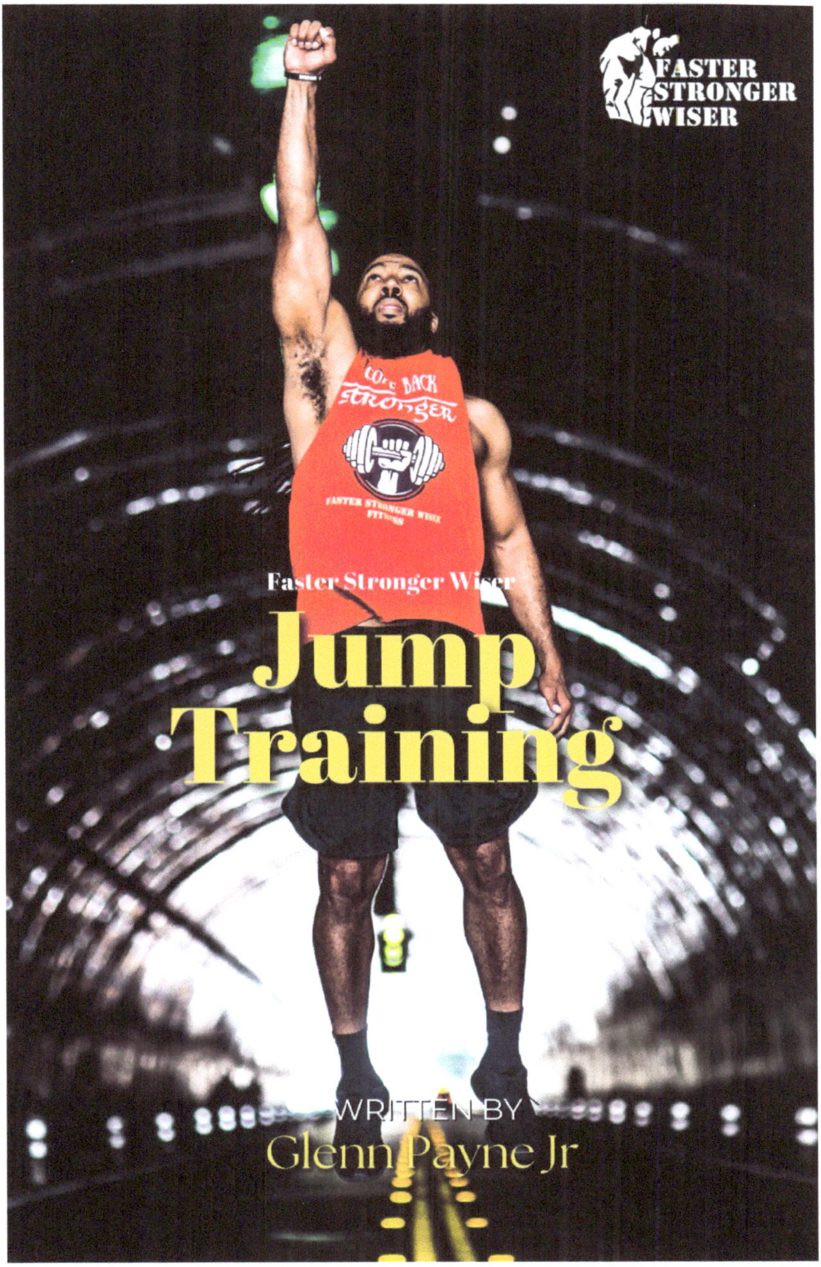

Faster Stronger Wiser Fitness

Faster Stronger Wiser Jump Training Program

Created by Glenn Payne Jr.

NASM, AFAA Certified Trainer

Precision Nutrition Level 1 Coach

Spartan SGX Coach

For more routines visit

Fasterstrongerwiser.com

This 10-day workout continues the Hectic Hundreds Jump Training Program and significantly increases your vertical leap, jump distance, and speed.

Sample Calendar						
Mon	**Tues**	**Wed**	**Thurs**	**Fri**	**Sat**	**Sun**
Day 1 Jump Height	**Day 2** Jump Distance	**Day 3** Jump Speed	**Day 4** Jump Power	**Day 5** All Around Jump Master	Rest Day 1	Rest Day 2
Day 6 Jump Height	**Day 7** Jump Distance	**Day 8** Jump Speed	**Day 9** Jump Power	**Day 10** All Around Jump Master	Rest Day 1	Rest Day 2

Before you get started.

Have a towel and water available because you will sweat a lot. This workout program is also part of The Hero Training Program, a 100-day full-body transformation program.

Disclaimer:

The exercises featured in this workout program are intense, so consult your physician before joining any fitness class or workout hosted by Faster Stronger Wiser Fitness and Glenn Payne Jr.

Faster Stronger Wiser Fitness and Glenn Payne Jr are not responsible for any injuries, sickness, or death from participating in this workout program.

Equipment Needed

Dumbbells (Various sizes)	Plyo Boxes	Fitness Bench

Table of Contents

The Hectic Hundreds Rep System

The Hectic Hundreds Rep System will help you achieve both strength and power in a short amount of time. This process is not based on science but on simple practice. In fitness, we don't see working out as exercise practice; we only see it as necessary to get stronger. When we switch our minds to treat our workouts as practice, we can apply an athlete's mindset to any exercise routine.

For example, a great shooter in basketball takes thousands of shots daily to master the art of shooting a basketball. The same goes for a boxer who practices his punches daily to stay sharp for his fights; if you were to treat exercise like you were practicing for a sport, you would develop a mastery of your body that will make you stronger than you ever thought you could be.

The Hectic Hundreds Rep System operates in three phases, but for this program, you will only utilize two phases.

The Hectic Hundreds Rules

1. Move up weight after 100 reps.
2. Start light.
3. Move up slowly.

Each rep system is progressive and designed to ensure you do not plateau in your workout. A workout plateau is where you stop seeing results in your routine, even though you are training with the same intensity.

These rep systems are primarily designed to be done with weight, but they can also be applied to bodyweight exercises to complete more advanced versions of the exercise, such as a push-up progressed to a clap push-up.

I will review how to track your progress to know when you should re-adjust your goals to ensure you get stronger.

HH Rep System 1: The Hectic Hundreds 4 Quarters

The Hectic Hundreds 4 Quarters is precisely what the rep system's title says. It's four quarters of work, 25 reps for four sets. This rep system is excellent because it lets you quickly get reps using lighter weights. The tempo used in this rep system is 1:1, which means 1 starts the rep, 0 seconds hold, and 1 completes the rep. For example, during a push-up, you would drop down for 1 second, hold for 0 seconds, then push yourself back to the starting point for 1 second. The purpose of this rep system is to flow through each rep while maintaining proper form.

The challenge in this rep system is completing the 25 reps without stopping. This phase is where you develop strength, and it's not about ego lifting. As you transition through this phase, you will gain enough strength to move on to the next training phase.

4 Sets: 25 Reps
Tempo: 1:0:1

HH Rep System 2: The Hectic Hundreds Double Trouble

This rep system lets you combine high and low repetitions to create a workout that builds strength and power without spending hours in the gym. This was one of my go-to systems in 30-minute sessions because we got to push through 4 to 5 exercises fast while using a decent amount of weight. This rep system is also good for transitioning to higher weights in the middle of a routine since the reps are lower in the last few sets.

This rep system consists of 8 sets, with the reps dropping by five after every two sets. The tempo used for this rep system will be a 1:2:1 cadence. The 2-second pause in the middle will allow more strength and stability to develop throughout the exercise. Jump training does not utilize pause reps, so that you will default most exercises to the 1:0:1 cadence.

Set 1: 20 Reps	**Set 5: 10 Reps**
Set 2: 20 Reps	**Set 6: 10 Reps**
Set 3: 15 Reps	**Set 7: 5 Reps**
Set 4: 15 Reps	**Set 8: 5 Reps**
Tempo: 1:2:1	

Note: This routine uses exercises that are timed and not rep-based. All the timed exercises will be placed after the rep-based exercises to ensure the routine flows smoothly.

Modifications

There will be no modifications in this routine; if an exercise feels too challenging, feel free to lower the weight, but there will be no substitutions for any exercise in this program. The goal is to master the workout; sometimes, you must step outside your comfort zone to achieve mastery. It's OK if there are exercises that cannot be completed immediately, but do your best to complete the routine.

Check out The Hectic Hundreds Stability Training to use as a builder routine for this workout program if there are exercises that you cannot complete.

Track Your Progress

You will only know if this program works if you track your progress. Five fitness tests will be conducted throughout this program to indicate how your body is progressing visually. Results will vary and can be affected through a solid nutrition regimen. This program does not offer nutrition advice or recommendations.

Use these statistics to track your progress throughout this program and see how your body changes from an aesthetic and performance viewpoint.

Body Statistics: Weight, Body Fat% and Measurements

The Faster Stronger Wiser Fitness Test

As well as the measurements and body fat%, the ability to master your body weight is a testament to your overall fitness level. The Faster Stronger Wiser Fitness test is based on timed bodyweight exercises. The full body weight test is 12 minutes long, and the entire test closes with a 1-mile run for time, which can be done outdoors or on a treadmill.

(Pro tip. Try to use the same running method each time to measure your progress better.)

On the next page, there are three fitness tests. Each one should be completed after completing the full Body Weight Blast Program.

Body Stats

	Test #1 Complete before starting the program.	Test #2 Complete after Week One	Test #3 Complete after Week Two
Date			
Weight			
Body Fat %			
Measurements			
Chest			
Waist			
Hips			
Right Arm			
Left Arm			
Right Leg			
Left Leg			

Fitness Tests

	Test #1 Complete before starting the program.	Test #2 Complete after Week One	Test #3 Complete after Week Two
Date			
Max Push Ups 3 Mins			
	Rest 1 Minute		
Max Pull Ups 3 Mins			
	Rest 1 Minute		
Max Squats 3 Mins			
	Rest 1 Minute		
Max Burpees 3 Mins			
	Rest 1 Minute		
1 Mile Run Time			

Faster Stronger Wiser Fitness

Week One

Each day will feel tough because of the number of reps necessary to complete the workout. Focus on maintaining your form throughout each exercise. Take time to complete the warmup and ensure you finish the cool down to complete the workout.

Close your eyes as you perform each exercise to add intensity to the workout.

Rest Days

Take a cold shower for 3-5 minutes daily to reduce your recovery time. This routine will work muscles that you haven't used before. Use these days to recover for the next week.

Day 1: Jump Height

This jump workout focuses on increasing jump height using dumbbells and barbells and is designed to enhance explosive power and generate force for higher vertical leaps. Dumbbells and barbells add resistance to your jump training, helping you build strength in the muscles involved in jumping.

Hero Training Warmup (Complete in a circuit)				
	Exercise	**Sets**	**Reps**	**Tempo**
1	Shoulder Tap to Superman	2	10	1:1:1
2	Split Stance Walk Out Combo	2	10	1:1:1

Workout (Complete in a circuit)					
	Exercise	**Sets**	**Reps**	**Tempo**	**Weight**
1	Barbell Squats	4	25	1:0:1	
2	Dumbbell Box Jumps	4	25	1:0:1	
3	Dumbbell Lateral Flying Step Ups	4	25 Each Side	1:0:1	
4	Dumbbell Forward Flying Step Ups	4	25 Each Side	1:0:1	
5	Burpees	4	25	1:0:1	

Hero Training Cool Down				
	Exercise	**Sets**	**Reps**	**Tempo**
1	Split Stance Walk Out Combo	1	10	1:1:1

Day 2: Jump Distance

This is a jump workout designed to increase jump distance. Dumbbells and Barbells are geared toward improving horizontal power and enhancing your ability to cover greater distances with each jump. The stairs will allow for a better workout and add to the development of the leg muscles.

	Hero Training Warmup (Complete in a circuit)			
	Exercise	**Sets**	**Reps**	**Tempo**
1	Shoulder Tap to Superman	2	10	1:1:1
2	Split Stance Walk Out Combo	2	10	1:1:1

	Workout (Complete in a circuit)				
	Exercise	**Sets**	**Reps**	**Tempo**	**Weight**
1	Barbell Lunges	4	25 Each Side	1:0:1	
2	Bounds	4	25	1:0:1	
3	Dumbbell Two-Foot Forward Hops	4	25 Each Side	1:0:1	
4	Dumbbell Two-Foot Lateral Hops	4	25 Each Side	1:0:1	
5	Stair Bounds	4	25	1:0:1	

	Hero Training Cool Down			
	Exercise	**Sets**	**Reps**	**Tempo**
1	Split Stance Walk Out Combo	1	10	1:1:1

Day 3: Jump Speed

This is a jump workout that emphasizes jump speed. This workout enhances your ability to generate force quickly and perform explosive, rapid jumps. This workout targets power and speed, which is especially beneficial for sports and activities requiring swift and explosive movements.

Hero Training Warmup (Complete in a circuit)				
	Exercise	**Sets**	**Reps**	**Tempo**
1	Shoulder Tap to Superman	2	10	1:1:1
2	Split Stance Walk Out Combo	2	10	1:1:1
Workout (Complete in a circuit)				
	Exercise	**Sets**	**Reps**	**Tempo**	**Weight**
1	Squat Jumps	4	25	1:0:1	
2	Jumping Jacks	4	25	1:0:1	
3	2 Foot Stair Hops	4	25	1:0:1	
4	1 Foot Stair Hops	4	25 Each Side	1:0:1	
5	Squat Jacks	4	25	1:0:1	
Hero Training Cool Down				
	Exercise	**Sets**	**Reps**	**Tempo**
1	Split Stance Walk Out Combo	1	10	1:1:1

Day 4: Jump Power

This is a jump workout designed to generate power using dumbbells and barbells. This workout is a dynamic training routine focusing on building explosive strength, maximizing vertical leap, and enhancing your ability to generate force rapidly.

Hero Training Warmup (Complete in a circuit)				
	Exercise	**Sets**	**Reps**	**Tempo**
1	Shoulder Tap to Superman	2	10	1:1:1
2	Split Stance Walk Out Combo	2	10	1:1:1

Workout (Complete in a circuit)				
	Exercise	**Sets**	**Reps**	**Tempo**	**Weight**
1	Barbell Squats	4	25	1:0:1	
2	Barbell Calf Raises	4	25	1:0:1	
3	Tuck Jumps	4	25	1:0:1	
4	Stair Lunges	4	25	1:0:1	
5	Stair Bounds	4	25	1:0:1	

Hero Training Cool Down				
	Exercise	**Sets**	**Reps**	**Tempo**
1	Split Stance Walk Out Combo	1	10	1:1:1

Day 5: All Around Jump Master

This comprehensive jump workout targets every muscle group used for jumping. This workout is essential for developing your explosive power, agility, and overall jumping performance. It engages the legs, core, and upper body muscles to maximize your vertical leap and athleticism.

Hero Training Warmup (Complete in a circuit)				
	Exercise	**Sets**	**Reps**	**Tempo**
1	Shoulder Tap to Superman	2	10	1:1:1
2	Split Stance Walk Out Combo	2	10	1:1:1

Workout (Complete in a circuit)					
	Exercise	**Sets**	**Reps**	**Tempo**	**Weight**
1	2 Foot Stair Hops	4	25	1:0:1	
2	Burpees	4	25	1:0:1	
3	Squat Jumps	4	25	1:0:1	
4	Jump Lunges	4	25 Each Side	1:0:1	
5	Goblet Grip Squats	4	25	1:0:1	

Hero Training Cool Down				
	Exercise	**Sets**	**Reps**	**Tempo**
1	Split Stance Walk Out Combo	1	10	1:1:1

Week Two

This week focuses on changing the rep system to give your body a different feel from the routine. The routine is completed in a circuit, so ensure that you complete the exercises in order and follow the rep system to get the best results. For example:

Set 1 will be 20 reps for each exercise except for timed exercises.

Set 2 will be 20 Reps for each exercise except for timed exercises.

Set 3 will be 15 reps for each exercise except for timed exercises.

Set 4 will be 15 reps for each exercise except for timed exercises.

Set 5 will be ten reps for each exercise except for timed exercises.

Set 6 will be ten reps for each exercise except for timed exercises.

Set 7 will be five reps for each exercise except for timed exercises.

Set 8 will be five reps for each exercise except for timed exercises.

Rest Days

Take a cold shower for 3-5 minutes daily to reduce your recovery time. This routine will work muscles that you haven't used before. Use these days to recover for the next week.

Day 6: Jump Height II

This day repeats day one but uses a different rep system to challenge your body differently.

	Hero Training Warmup (Complete in a circuit)			
	Exercise	**Sets**	**Reps**	**Tempo**
1	Shoulder Tap to Superman	2	10	1:1:1
2	Split Stance Walk Out Combo	2	10	1:1:1
	Workout (Complete in a circuit)			
	Exercise	**Sets & Reps**	**Tempo**	**Weight**
1	Barbell Squats	2 Sets of 20 Reps	1:0:1	
2	Dumbbell Box Jumps		1:0:1	
3	Dumbbell Lateral Flying Step Ups (Both Sides)	2 Sets of 15 Reps	1:0:1	
		2 Sets of 10 Reps		
4	Dumbbell Forward Flying Step Ups (Both Sides)	2 Sets of 5 Reps	1:0:1	
5	Burpees		1:0:1	
	Hero Training Cool Down			
	Exercise	**Sets**	**Reps**	**Tempo**
1	Split Stance Walk Out Combo	1	10	1:1:1

Day 7: Jump Distance

This day repeats day two but uses a different rep system to challenge your body differently.

	Hero Training Warmup (Complete in a circuit)			
	Exercise	**Sets**	**Reps**	**Tempo**
1	Shoulder Tap to Superman	2	10	1:1:1
2	Split Stance Walk Out Combo	2	10	1:1:1

	Workout (Complete in a circuit)			
	Exercise	**Sets & Reps**	**Tempo**	**Weight**
1	Barbell Lunges (Both Sides)	2 Sets of 20 Reps	1:0:1	
2	Bounds	2 Sets of 15 Reps	1:0:1	
3	Dumbbell Two-Foot Forward Hops (Both Sides)	2 Sets of 10 Reps	1:0:1	
4	Dumbbell Two-Foot Lateral Hops (Both Sides)	2 Sets of 5 Reps	1:0:1	
5	Stair Bounds		1:0:1	

	Hero Training Cool Down			
	Exercise	**Sets**	**Reps**	**Tempo**
1	Split Stance Walk Out Combo	1	10	1:1:1

Day 8: Jump Speed

This day repeats day three but uses a different rep system to challenge your body differently.

	Hero Training Warmup (Complete in a circuit)			
	Exercise	**Sets**	**Reps**	**Tempo**
1	Shoulder Tap to Superman	2	10	1:1:1
2	Split Stance Walk Out Combo	2	10	1:1:1

	Workout (Complete in a circuit)			
	Exercise	**Sets & Reps**	**Tempo**	**Weight**
1	Squat Jumps	2 Sets of 20 Reps	1:0:1	
2	Jumping Jacks		1:0:1	
3	2 Foot Stair Hops	2 Sets of 15 Reps	1:0:1	
4	1 Foot Stair Hops (Both Sides)	2 Sets of 10 Reps	1:0:1	
5	Squat Jacks	2 Sets of 5 Reps	1:0:1	

	Hero Training Cool Down			
	Exercise	**Sets**	**Reps**	**Tempo**
1	Split Stance Walk Out Combo	1	10	1:1:1

Day 9: Jump Power

This day repeats day four but uses a different rep system to challenge your body differently.

	Hero Training Warmup (Complete in a circuit)			
	Exercise	**Sets**	**Reps**	**Tempo**
1	Shoulder Tap to Superman	2	10	1:1:1
2	Split Stance Walk Out Combo	2	10	1:1:1

	Workout (Complete in a circuit)			
	Exercise	**Sets & Reps**	**Tempo**	**Weight**
1	Barbell Squats	2 Sets of 20 Reps	1:0:1	
2	Barbell Calf Raises		1:0:1	
3	Tuck Jumps	2 Sets of 15 Reps	1:0:1	
4	Stair Lunges	2 Sets of 10 Reps	1:0:1	
5	Stair Bounds		1:0:1	
		2 Sets of 5 Reps		

	Hero Training Cool Down			
	Exercise	**Sets**	**Reps**	**Tempo**
1	Split Stance Walk Out Combo	1	10	1:1:1

Day 10: All Around Jump Master

This day repeats day five but uses a different rep system to challenge your body differently.

Hero Training Warmup (Complete in a circuit)			
Exercise	**Sets**	**Reps**	**Tempo**
1 Shoulder Tap to Superman	2	10	1:1:1
2 Split Stance Walk Out Combo	2	10	1:1:1

Workout (Complete in a circuit)			
Exercise	**Sets & Reps**	**Tempo**	**Weight**
1 2 Foot Stair Hops	2 Sets of 20 Reps	1:0:1	
2 Burpees		1:0:1	
3 Squat Jumps	2 Sets of 15 Reps	1:0:1	
4 Jump Lunges (Both Sides)	2 Sets of 10 Reps	1:0:1	
5 Goblet Grip Squats	2 Sets of 5 Reps	1:0:1	

Hero Training Cool Down			
Exercise	**Sets**	**Reps**	**Tempo**
1 Split Stance Walk Out Combo	1	10	1:1:1

FSW Jump Training Exercise List
Hero Training Warmup & Cool Down

Shoulder Taps to Superman

Start in a plank position with your hands under your shoulders and your feet hip-width apart. Tap your shoulders with each hand, then lower yourself to the ground. Next, extend your arms in front of your body and lift your chest, arms, and legs off the ground as if you were flying. Return to the plank position.

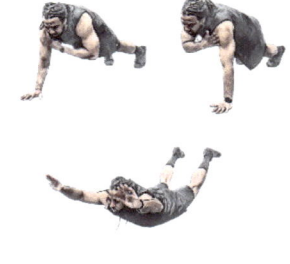

Split Stance Walk Out Combo

Start with your feet hip-width apart. Next, bend forward until your hands touch the ground. Walk your hands out until you are in a cobra stretch. Focus on pressing your hips into the ground for 3 seconds. Next, release the stretch and touch your toes, going right hand to left toe and left hand to right toe. Return to the starting point and swing your arms above your head. Repeat the drill.

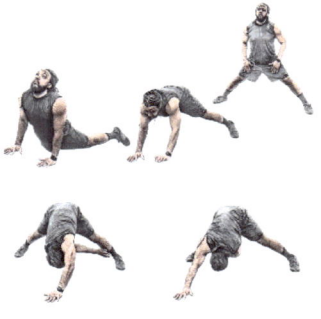

Day 1: Jump Height

Barbell Squats

Start standing with your feet shoulder-width apart in front of a plyo box. Grab a dumbbell in each hand. Swing your arms down, bend your knees, and jump onto the plyo box. Land softly by bending your knees as you land. Step back down to restart the exercise.

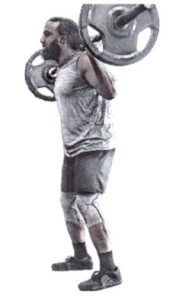
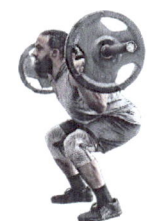

Dumbbell Box Jumps

Start standing with your feet shoulder-width apart in front of a plyo box and a dumbbell in each hand. Swing your arms down, bend your knees, and jump onto the plyo box. Land softly by bending your knees as you land. Step back down to restart the exercise.

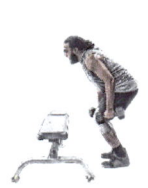
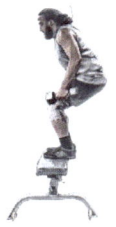

Dumbbell Flying Lateral Step-Ups

Start standing before a plyo box or a bench with a dumbbell in each hand. Step up onto the plyo box laterally and explode into the air. Switch legs in midair and land on the opposite leg. Repeat on the opposite side.

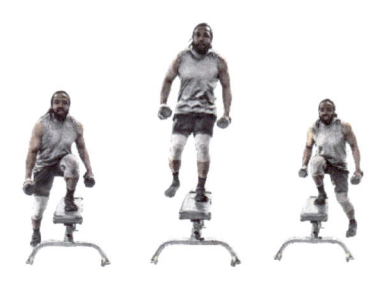

Dumbbell Flying Forward Step Ups

Start standing before a plyo box or bench with a dumbbell in each hand. Step up onto the plyo box and explode into the air. Switch legs in midair and land on the opposite leg. Repeat on the opposite side.

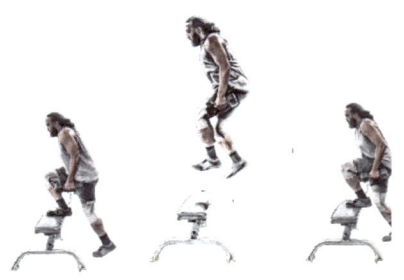

Burpees

Start standing with your feet hip-width apart and bend your knees. Jump up into the air and touch your toes by pulling your feet up in front of you—land softly by bending your knees upon landing.

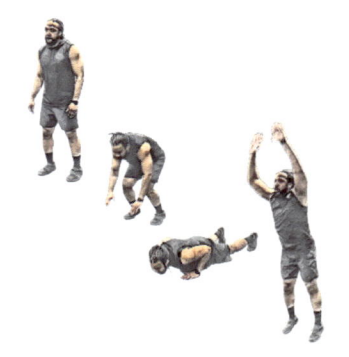

Day 2: Jump Distance

Barbell Lunges

Step forward with one leg, lowering your body until both knees are bent at 90-degree angles, with your front knee aligned with your ankle and your back knee hovering just above the ground. Push through your front heel to return to the starting position. Repeat on the opposite side.

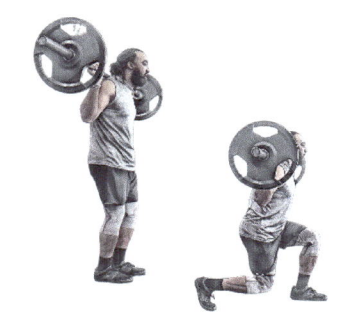

Bounds

Start with your feet hip-width apart. Lift your arms and wing them downwards. Bend your knees and jump forward as far as you can—land softly by bending your knees upon landing.

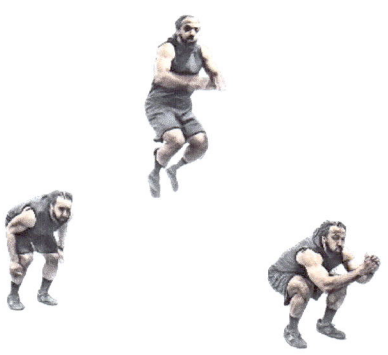

Dumbbell Two-Foot Forward Hops

Start with your feet hip-width apart and a dumbbell in each hand. Bend your knees and jump forward, then backward. Land softly by bending your knees as you land.

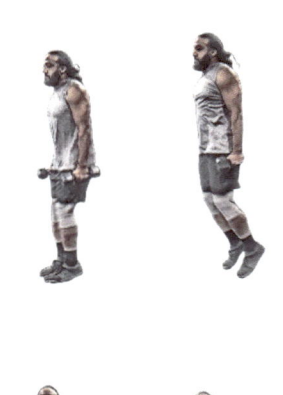

Dumbbell Lateral Two Foot Hops

Start with your feet hip-width apart and a dumbbell in each hand. Bend your knees and jump laterally to the side. Land softly by bending your knees as you land.

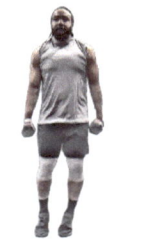
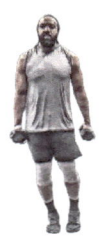

Stair Bounds

Start standing at the bottom of the stairs with your legs shoulder-width apart. Jump up 3 to 4 steps until you reach the top. Walk back down the stairs and repeat the exercise.

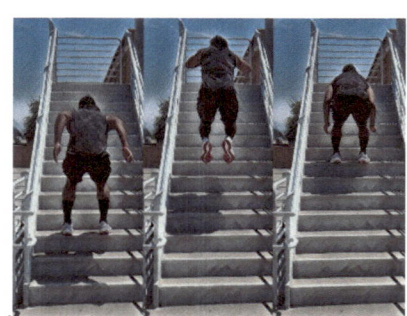

Day 3: Jump Speed

Squat Jumps

Start with your feet hip-width apart. Bend your knees and jump off the ground. Land softly by bending your knees as you land.

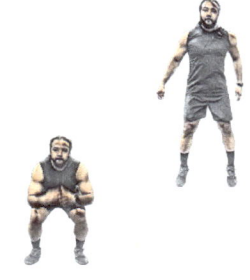

Jumping Jacks

Start with your feet hip-width apart and hands down by your side. Jump out and extend your hands over your head. Return to the starting position.

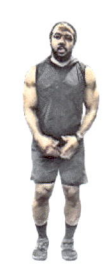
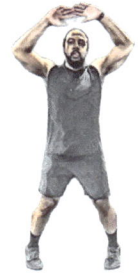

2 Foot Stair Hops

Start standing before a plyo box with a dumbbell in each hand. Step up onto the plyo box laterally and explode into the air. Switch legs in midair and land on the opposite leg. Repeat on the opposite side.

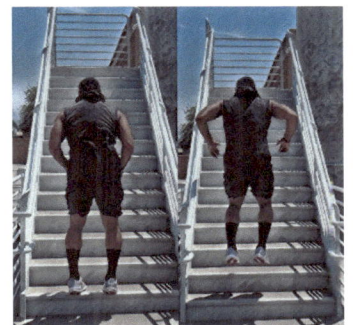

One Foot Stair Hops

Start standing at the bottom of the stairs with your legs shoulder-width apart. Stand onto one leg, then jump up each step until you reach the top. Walk back down the stairs and repeat the exercise on the other leg.

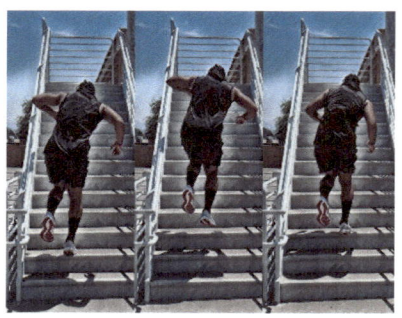

Squat Jacks

Start with your feet shoulder-width apart. Drop into a squat, jump into a close squat stance (feet together), and then jump back to the starting position. Keep your chest up the entire time.

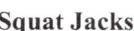
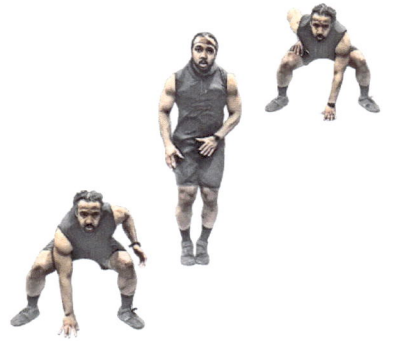

Day 4: Jump Power

Barbell Squats

Start with a barbell on the meaty part of your back. Position your feet shoulder-width apart and turn your feet outwards. Drop into a squat by lowering your body to a 90-degree angle. Squeeze your glutes to rise back to the top.

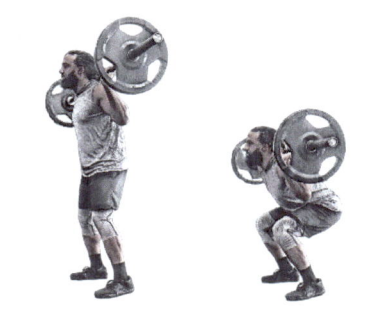

Barbell Calf Raises

Start with a barbell on the meaty part of your back. Place your feet hip-width apart and lift your heels off the ground until you are on your toes. Lower back to the ground and repeat.

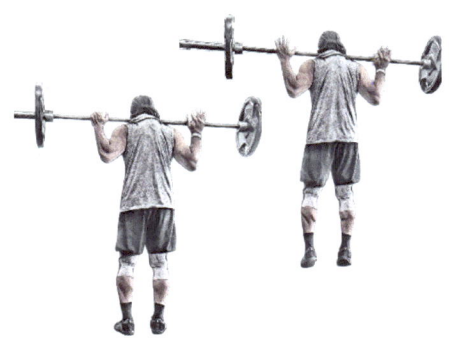

Tuck Jumps

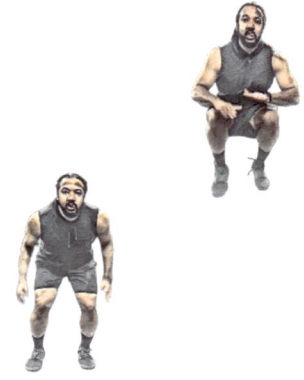

Start with your feet hip-width apart. Lift your arms and wing them downwards. Bend your knees and jump into the air as high as you can. Pull your knees up to your chest and land softly, bending your knees upon landing.

Stair Lunges

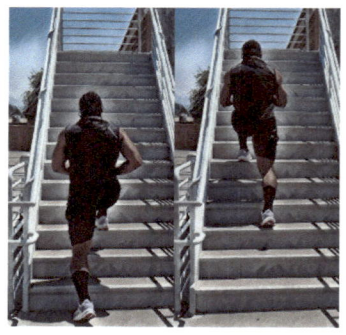

Start standing at the bottom of the stairs with your legs shoulder-width apart. Turn to the side and step up 2- 3 steps until you reach the top. Walk back down the stairs and repeat the exercise on the opposite side.

Stair Bounds

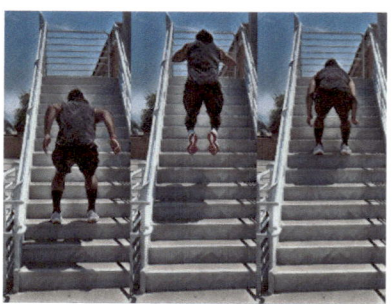

Start standing at the bottom of the stairs with your legs shoulder-width apart. Jump up 3 to 4 steps until you reach the top. Walk back down the stairs and repeat the exercise.

Day 5: All Around Jump Master

2 Foot Stair Hops

Start standing at the bottom of the stairs with your legs shoulder-width apart. Jump up each step until you reach the top. Walk back down the stairs and repeat the exercise.

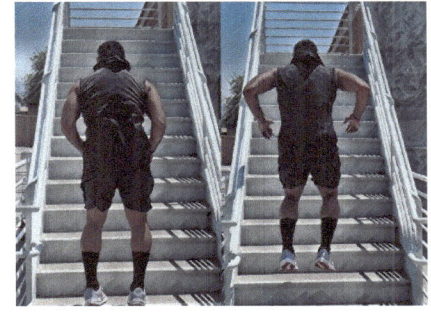

Burpees

Place your hands on the floor. Hop back, bringing your body to the ground. Hop forward, landing, and standing straight up. Increase speed as you feel comfortable.

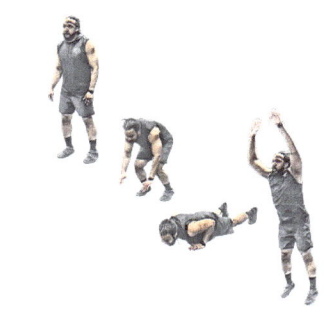

Squat Jumps

Start with your feet hip-width apart. Bend your knees and jump off the ground. Land softly by bending your knees as you land.

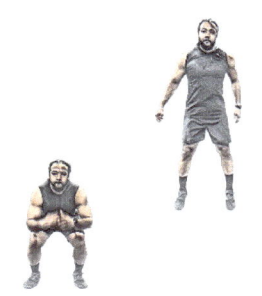

Jump Lunges

Start with feet together. Jump one foot back and the other forward, lowering until the knees are 90 degrees. Quickly jump your back foot forward and front foot back.

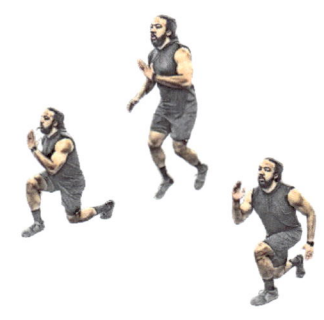

Goblet Grip Squats

Grab a dumbbell and hold it in a goblet grip position. Drop down into a squat. Squeeze your glutes to push yourself back up to the starting position.

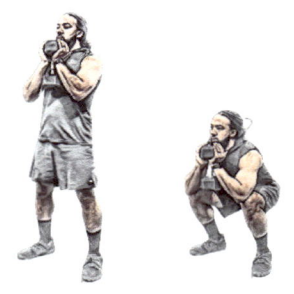

Thank You

Thank you for challenging yourself with this workout program.
This is one portion of the FSW Jump Training Program.

www.ingramcontent.com/pod-product-compliance
Lightning Source LLC
Chambersburg PA
CBHW050858290526
45792CB00002B/651